Out in the Dark:
a queer road to mental health

ISBN: 978-1-998061-11-2

Copyright © 2023 Suzan Digh

All rights reserved.

Cover Art by Suzan Digh

To my wife. I am so glad to have found you.

Contents

Introduction 4
A Little Crazy 6
The Falling 36
Treatment 61
Seeking 85
Abuses 99
Coming Out 123
Just Plain Queer 132
The Rising 148

Introduction

This is a collection of Found poetry wherein the poet erases or blacks out (redacts) the bulk of the words on a page and the words that remain are used to create poetry; these remaining words appear in the poems in the same sequence as in the original text.

The source document is an early draft version of my recently completed (as yet unpublished) creative non-fiction novel which explores the mental health issues that surrounded my coming out as queer, and my subsequent struggles with acceptance, medical interventions, sexuality, drugs, and alcohol.

In this book the words do retain their original order, however, capitalization, punctuation, and line spacing have been modified in many of the poems.

The poems' titles consist of a number (and letter) representing the order the poem came out of the source document, and whether it was a digital blackout (B) or an erasure (E). I left many of the erased poems in their original shape on the page, with the spacing as it appeared. In some cases there was more than one poem per page, and those are marked with a small letter (i.e. 70b).

The poems have been arranged in chapters so the poems will be out of numerical sequence. If there is a poem number missing, it is because that poem was edited out of the collection before publication.

* * *

Some of these poems have been previously published in "Another Dark Place" where the image of the source document was included. In this collection I have not included any of the source document's blacked out images so it will read more like a traditional poetry book.

And, the final note is… this collection is very dark. Mental health struggles are real, and the source novel explores some very dark experiences, so it is not unexpected that the poetry stemming from that text reflects this darkness.

There is light at the end, we just have to get there.

A Little Crazy

23.

morning,
dark, empty

I talk, but the echo - loud -
in my mind.

My voice feels strange,
different from mine.

85b.

I stand in the rain.
People smile, meaningless —
    some with auras.

I stare through averted eyes;
they seem ordinary.

A raindrop lands,
the dark spot spreads.

91.

I shudder at the thought:
   (never fully erased)
I had already been destroyed.

A pressure builds.
I swallow it and…

I snap.

85c.

I sometimes just feel like screaming.

I'm tired.

Wondering why I excuse myself,
my friend laughed and said I was weird.

85.

An older lady
   — her voice calms me —
   — I can't feel my slap —

didn't feel anything…

82.

I tell myself I am content.
Still, in my drink…

a strange physical urge.

81c.

She backs out of the direction she had been going.
She didn't know I was easy,
and could be flattered.

She should know of my frequent disconnections,

   perhaps.

Not elaborating, I pretend to be normal.

79b.

Even those who hear voices have the right to feel how life passes.

78.

I am paranoid.
Something giggles…
    unnoticeably.

71.

Blank.
Worry tickles the back of my neck.

Yank.
I run, angry.

Plop.
I shake, relaxing.

Forced…
having lost all.

68.

A little voice whispers that I'd die with the passion.

    I fall back onto the bed with…
        …hands touching my body
        …my lover's kisses on my face
    My lover moans softly and…

I wipe the tears off my cheeks.

63c.

Mopping the kitchen floor,
I avoid the kitchen.

I peel off my wet clothes —
wanting knocks quietly.

Partly open,
I touch myself.

62b.

She picks quickly —
wishing her selection would choose privacy.

Some young girls work,
for several dollars, on the sidewalk.

It is dark and wet and eerie.

Close — for a moment—
I stop at the edge of illegality.

62.

I plant myself and wait for the door to close.

I feel dirty,
wrong to watch her as I am,
to invade her privacy.

I accept it is possible to invade someone.

48.

        I retrace my steps   if I was thinking,
it fades.
I kneel beside my secret.   The secret
- it's much too big -   but I keep
it. I would confide   to a friend - if I had one.

Nobody   looks into my secret -
always much too busy drinking   cheap wine, and my
mother believes in privacy.

47.

  I find myself in the bathroom. I look into   the mirror and
see nothing. I guess
this doesn't bother me.   I have
disappeared and I don't worry.

 I flush the toilet   so my mother
don't start wondering
that I really expect them to notice me -
I am not visible   not important
- during the daylight hours.

46.

I don't think   words leave my throat.   They get stuck between my teeth.   I've forgotten   I want to yell at him.

42b.

Flesh -
   permeates.

That smell -
   familiar.

A man -
   reaching across me.

Very nice -
   I try resistance.

She promised I wouldn't have this fear.

She lied.

33.

I check the stress.

It doubled - an ocean -
- a distance -
everywhere.

I recede.

E11.

                        Watching   comfort
scream   I laugh —
           so stupid,   crying for things
that don't exist.   I would
                be better off
foolish.

30.

the cold floor against my back
the world, out of focus
(whose eyes am I looking through?)
Scared, I laugh.

27.

Untie me,
somebody talk to me.

Make sense!

I'll follow it.

25.

(senryu)

what is wrong with me?
I move, I strain, I flex, but
panic enlarges.

18.

Willing to listen,
can you hear?
Nice. Glad.

An old hinge
creaking? Go complain.
Don't think. Don't worry.

7.

My mind splits,
    slowly.

I find the mirror.
I'm not disappeared.

I don't think, still, I
can never really be sure.

8.

My mother couldn't possibly be content,
only hidden, like something cold.

I worry,
wondering what secret they'd touch

89.

We wanted to die —
we thought.

She was surprised I thought she would kill me.
I explained that way was as good as any.

She laughed and said I was weird.

B6.

I walk along the river, alone.
I know this can't seem happy.

I want love but I don't have time.

Crying on the bank of the river, I tell myself these pleasant moments can
kill.

It hurts to expect more.

70.

Trouble prickles.

She identifies herself.

I am too busy to hear her explain—
a ringing stupid explanation.

Incoherency continues.

The conversation, more logical,
does ease my mind.

I have gone home.

The Falling

67.

On the edge, just older than a child,
I ran away from tortures.

Alone and dreaming of laughter,
I wonder how to explain I know better.

Sober (*I don't want to be*),
and too broke to afford snort.

84.

My head aches and I can't get up.
I spent all day struggling to hold reason.

A woman is standing, sock feet,
watching, concerned.
A man is studying two girls behind me.

They are hard,
and the words sound like lies.

83b.

Wet-cheeked, alone, I quietly unlock the door —
terrified, smiling.

Death is waiting patiently.
The light is empty.
I stagger on the verge.

83.

I roll over.
She is too pretty.
I touch her bottom lip, unsure.
Softly, she sighs.

My conscience alleviates its guilt,
slivers of pleasure slice within.

… Blood… on her arms.
I glance at the syringe on the table.
Her eyes are closed.
The ambulance arrives.
They scoop up the condemning note.

82c.

The polluted waves splash.
The rocks surge.

I step to freedom.
Shocking into non-existence,
the force weakens my body.
And I lose.

E22.

    Only seconds   for me to slip
away into the dark.

    And it   offers me
comfort   so I   quietly

                                                       strangle.

E7.

    Years later

                                    in   the depths

it's empty.   So numb.

The Falling

B3.

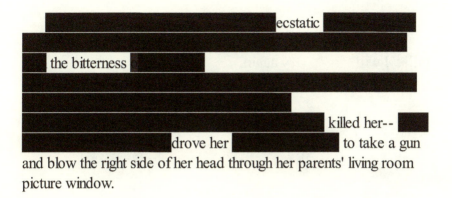

and blow the right side of her head through her parents' living room picture window.

—

Ecstatic,

the bitterness killed her.
Drove her to take a gun
and blow the right side of her head through her parents' living room window.

E1.

        I wake up. It is dark.
                                        There were not enough
pills. I will   try again.
                                   — beyond disappointment —

66b.

Tears build little castles in my throat.
Sorrow rages.

I will be overwhelmed and…

nobody will know.

65.

These choices fall
like some confining washroom stall.

I curl, programmed to regret my aloneness.

My heart begins to bleed.

The blood drops on my outheld hand.

I am left.

63b.

My body splattered
would make too big a mess for the rain to wash away.

I am not high enough for splashing.
The temptations loud.

63.

Control
    the lip,
    this great grey tongue,
    the eyes,
the temptation.
I ponder them for many minutes.

They offer empty promises.

56.

All these early risers -
always someplace, doing something.

Winter is soon. I shiver.

The washroom smells like a combo of soap and hairspray,
and is comfortably warm.

In the hot water, soaking my head,
I hear echoes through the porcelain.

Day in, day out, I struggle.

My head, the womb-warmth of the tub -
the confining walls,
    wrapping.

I open.
I gulp.
I must…

        water…

my throat…

50.
                              About six months
ago.   God forbade me to   feel nothing.
Unless I am able to cry, or yell, or fight, I would do nothing
but lay there,   feel nothing. So   God
believed me because He knows. I can't lie.
But I did lie, and now I have these little green pills to take
me away from this.

49.

I am distracted by   his wife.

I   listen.   Their voices make no sense to me.

                                        I wake up.   I am on my knees by my bed. My hand   wrapped around something round. My head is resting on my   neck.

          Voice is louder. They are talking.   I can't hear.

But I don't mind because I have this little round bottle stashed.

   The contents - little green pills - fall into a random pattern. I don't count them because I don't care how many there are. There are enough for me, and, if   not, I will collect more

 for next time. I am a patient woman.

          God

   love   me ?

41.

I played with emotion.
I pretended.
I lied.
I killed.

I took a gun -
I was supposed to die,
but it doesn't hurt.

Unbearable, I have no escape.

Falling into terror,
I can't break free.

20.

Her parents understand the cops and the hospital.
They thought trouble had been looking for me.

They began to question me - a girl.
"I used to go to her bedroom."…
    (they never took me as very insulted.)
"but the last time I had a friend, she died."

19.

Remove our eyes.
Blood stains in the hospital.

People overreact.
I stain the carpet.
They have bought a new one.

Her fault really,
she realized the pressure
and she didn't like it.

She didn't want to.

9b.

(senryu)

A strange noise. Thinking
I hear voices. Normal for
my paranoia.

3.

(senryu)

a random pattern
too many little green pills
it would do, long-term.

3b.

too many little green pills
the bed sags

they fill my mouth

I am too dry to swallow -
forced open

I faint.

11.

Psychotic coma
in complete darkness I read minds
and sometimes,
I scare people.

22.

I can't feel
I can't move.
I can't anything.

I faint.
I scream.
I wonder.

I wish.

I stand.
I stop.

Fade out…

Treatment

74.

I want my powerful
guiding doctor
to prescribe the appropriate medications.

I stupidly finger the pills,
my thought processes toxic.

I skip the prescribed.
I adjust the chosen pills.
I add to the mixture to see if they help relax.

E10.

I force myself to think about
> (*It only takes moments, in and out,
> like an assembly line*)

the seven others sitting in the lobby just outside,
waiting with anticipation.

I should be grateful.
There's not much to remember.
I will lose nothing significant with their electric current.

Calm now, I smile as they fasten the electrodes to my temples.

B4.

The ceiling on my grave —
　　many prefer wood.

The smell of sunned, dead meat—
　　stronger, penetrating.

The nurse wipes her perfume —
　　it is nice, the smell.

Treatment

B2.

█████ The chemicals █████ spread through my blood. █████████ climb up my neck, in bursts and spurts, with the beat of my heart. ████████████████████
█████ They spread, multiply, cover and coat █████ my thoughts. Slow, my mind fades. █████████
████████████████████These foreign agents burst within it. Wavy lines cross my vision and the float comes; it sweeps me up. ██████████████████████████

E9.

She intrudes on the nut ward —

  they monitor until they are sure I will behave
    appropriately,

    the pinprick her potent threat —

and then slips outside.

My arms become too long
and they are wrapped around her neck
and I can't untangle them.

And the men in white come.

E8.

     The ceiling is white.
        The bed is hard.   My arms are strapped down. Metal bars at the sides of the bed create thick lines in my vision.
           All this is strangely comforting.

E5.

    Anger   in great strong waves
tosses me about.   Humiliation makes me
   scream— but there is no sound   so I am
silent.

                                    My wonderful doctor
comes.   I
    try to ignore the sound of her
                                        sighs
of pleasure   and, just for a moment,
          I long to be free of all this
living.   .
                           I feel a pinprick.
    I guess   they have been kind enough to give me
another needle, so I won't cry anymore.

E4.

                      Moving from somewhere —
not within my   skull…   in someone else's?

                           The smack   connects.
              I lose my sight for a second —
then   the cold
floor.
              The world is   out of focus
                    wavy   like a
        tv with bad reception, a rolling screen of
characters.

                    The orderlies, two of them, pile on top.
          A needle comes out of someone's uniform pocket.

        And the chemical   enters my brain.

                          What?
     Nobody will tell me, even if I could
ask, so I guess that means I don't need to know.

E3.

Someone talking.
The words scratch my face,
just beyond my fingertips, somewhere over my head —
taunting me.

I search.
I will find them,
after all, I remember how painful it is.
I shove.
The pressure builds.
Escape burns and bounces through emptiness —
The gap between the outside world,
    I trust still exists?

The ache is something else.
Something hovers close.

I recognize my own voice in my ears,
my body, the IV, my arm…

Women in white uniforms, one in blue,
don't know I am helpless.

B1.

I slide back into my body.
It must be the medication.

They are monitoring me.
This is standard policy:
    docile, on the floor, getting needled.

The jabs don't even bother to look for a vein.
Maybe it doesn't matter.

51.

Shock treatments -   nothing against the psychiatric profession - make me calmer, and more open to say yes until after my doctor explained the memory damage.
                                                                        How I would lose -   would be damaged   -   I knew   would scare me into silence.

42.

Rotting flesh -
the smell permeates.

What is that smell?

Familiar faces:
    a nurse, feels good.
    a machine, ominous.
    a man talking, an orderly
        reaching across me.

I smell.

36.

The psychiatric medication -
teach me a lesson.

The straps wrapped around me,
    not in vain,
I begin to feel sane.

They have to hold me -
can never get out.

35.

In my arm,
another needle -
so I wouldn't cry anymore.

The chemicals race.

The ceiling is white.

31.

I feel the needle,
my veins betrayed,
but the chemicals gently explode
and I feel nothing.

———

Switch channels,
watch the multicolors.

Perfectly beautiful,
memories come easily.

26.

My eyes are closed,
I must be tied down.
They control me, I guess.

15.

Doctor wouldn't lie?
These voices -
don't see anyone there -
just my wonderful doctor.
I must be
very insecure.

14.

Final sensation.
No relief in a psychiatric ward.

Slipping into the woodwork,
you die.

12.

Obviously, the fact that the hospital
was really great
    - for a matter of minutes -
didn't shock people.

10.

I wake up.
The voices I hear worry about me -
my paranoia.

They are silly,
and I kinda resent
my medication.

9.

A strange noise
thinking I hear voices.
Normal for a change.

57.

Mood-stabilized,
Anti-psychoticized,
Forcibly anti-depressed…
I must take these pills.

I would rather be suppressed for the sake of peace.

Knowing my withdrawal is starting, I sit on the floor —
sink within my craving.

Dullness greets me.

73.

Murder, of all my options, can't clearly remain my choice.

I didn't really want to worry about being insane.
I can't embarrass myself if crazy?

Last time, my craziness made me realize I am illogical.

I never did want to be mental.
Next time, it could work — her cures.

Seeking

28.

I should have
the loneliness
not just in my body.

God has left me.

16.

The noise disturbed me
 - having a relapse -
my medication is very sweet,
my body, physical.

E21.

        I don't know her, don't care about her, don't desire her. But, inevitably,   we head off for her bed. I try   to have sex;
                her hands touch me and
                              I manage to stifle the screaming.   I make it through the motions and finally I'm   asleep.

E20.

Fucking her,
talking.   I'm shaking.

                        I don't know how

    to leave. She asks   to
sleep together and I   feel guilty
                and   politely refuse.
                                                                    I

    leave.

E18.

                    A woman —

                                      I
spill her drink down the front of her shirt; she will let me replace the drink.   I
        offer

      to help her change.
        We   go back to her apartment and take our shirts off.

E16.

                         I don't know how much later — days?   I find myself curled around somebody. I hope she doesn't mind my skin on hers.

          Love   ricochets around.

                                  I don't even know this woman I'm lying with

     in my own bedroom.

                                Or is that the other way around?

70b.

My pants drop.

The silence flows.

She is also coming, we both have.

We should talk…
I open my mouth, dumbly…

45.

I don't really

feel darkness cry out. I rise

slowly and realize

touching

me

** God **

He is still with me!

5.

Mostly he knew
living bothers me.

God comforts me.
I feel better.
Fading,
God rests.

4.

Woman coughs,
    smokes
    dies.

Nighttime again.

Calmer,
God explained.

4b.

(senryu)

Woman coughs, smokes, dies.
Nighttime again. Calmer, God
explained: feel better.

43.

She's very nice,
if only she would come closer.
I try to get her attention but meet resistance.

She promised I wouldn't have to betray
this fear.

She lied.

E15.

I stand, cut off.

I feel low.

I know that situation is trivial.

The dark night isn't silent.
I listen to the noises of God.

I cry.

Abuses

6.

His tongue
down my throat.
I am too dry to take any more.
They fill my mouth.
I swallow.

Forced open,
I faint.

The bed sags.

21.

I neck with
my nice constant care nurse.

They took him away.

29.

Loud and long, against my will,
moving in the bed.

Stop!

58.

I oblige him,
while he is relieving himself.

By the time I am clothed, he is at the top of the stairs,
smoking.

24.

Whomever you are touching me,
always in the same place,
and I try
    - I imagine -
to scratch.

Abuses

E2.

                        The bed is different.

Who is touching me?   It
doesn't hurt. I   pull
                left   but   can't
                        go away.

                            I   imagine
                  this strange bed.
                       My face itches; I try to
scratch but my arm won't
                             move.

         Panic floats.
            Someone is doing this.
                  I can't stop   it -
                            let me free!

87.

He tries to kiss me.
I pull my head back.

He continues —
pushes me against the door and runs his hands along my breasts.

I scream.

He unbuttons his jeans.
He grunts.

He says it's only to please me,
that he knows I just don't want to admit it.

He comes,
and flops back against the seat on his side of the car.

He drives silently,
and drops me off at the corner.

I fold memory
and nothing ever happened.

86.

I faint,
amazed how small my memory.
I lose focus and
he says he knows a nice place.
He is sure I'm interested.

He explains it is much better,
the second go
and plans out the third.

My head is fuzzy.
I am amazed.

I laugh, thinking him joking.

B7.

Male, screaming —
he begs.
He's scared.

I was too, the first time.

(Don't think of it —
I'll want to end the squealing male screaming.)

53.

My eyes are forced open by contractions somewhere behind my forehead.

          I   hear   footsteps   -
pain is fading, distant.   The bed
sags beside me.   His hand
rests on my right breast. His breath reeks of alcohol.
My eyes are open.   I
lose my thoughts.   The world
is blank. I am blank.

          I feel a weight.   I feel breath
but my lips don't respond. I am scared that
I am not.

                                              The light fades.

77b.

I have a headache.
I reject her

    — an excuse

and slip two pills,
dry-mouthed.

79.

Later, I tell her I would rather not have to face the shakes.

We fill up drink glasses.
Mildly intoxicated, she must be joining.

I am amused,
and coherent enough.

I think about my doctor,
my medications, her advice.
I dislike her, distrust her.

I deserve to shake my dependency.

I am sane enough.

77.

The Prof asks if my drink is ok.
She seems concerned.

> — my drink a painkiller,
> and medicine —

I thank her and say she should
fill the glass up.

76.

Gurgling gin,
my audacity makes me smile.
My doctor says it will not mix with my medications.

I relax in the soft black couch.
I own my right to drink.

My hands fall to the couch beside me.
Feeling my alcohol —
I'm not sure I like it.

E19.

                                               Another drink...   I
wander   the edge of —   I don't know —

           some evil thing inside.

64b.

The closed windows filter the street noises.
I am uncomfortable.
I take a bottle from my night table drawer
    and slip several pills between my lips.

It is hard in the middle of the bed.

The wailing grows fainter.

E6.

The								blot—
			faster and faster and finally complete.
						Not even the unknown
returns.

59.

Conveniently,
I pour a depressing drink.

I am not allowed to — at least not this early in the day,
but,
I am in the depths of nothingness —
my semi-conscious body is freed from the grip,
briefly.

This desire ends, eventually —
these confining walls, burning.

I am grateful.

38.

I surrender to the chemical in my blood.

Quickly!

they burst.

95.

Her, shocked,
at the fact that I like a drink.

I leave the room,
— to drink—
trying to make myself comfortable.

She is looking through my fridge,
making a note…

I feel panicky.

I make sure she is still occupied,
before grabbing my bottle and dumping
into my mouth, head back.

I don't quite feel guilty for my chemical aids,
but I definitely feel something.

2.

I grasp my secret:
drinking
in privacy.
My head is loud.

Abuses

52.

    Yelling at the woman in the living room - she really is my wife, but one couldn't tell.
A wife.   Who needs a wife?
The yelling   bothers me.
The pressure   building,   slipping. I
cup   the palm of my hand,
sort of   rock slightly.
A very ugly

    slide down.   I am finished.
My mouth is   dry,
    bitter.   I swallow.
                                                                          I

close my eyes   to
   pain.

44.

It's not that bad.
It always feels better, after.

I'll feel better, after.

There's not much to remember, anyway.

Here I go.

Coming Out

81.

Phrasing made it possible for me to disappear
in this closet.

I fight its contents.

92.

Only I will get frustrated this evening.

    I have a date,
    and it excites me —
        I suspect love, no doubt.

    She, however,
    does not.

She makes me wonder if I am straight…

E14.

                                        She doesn't
          want   me   (she tells me).
                                       She isn't exactly lying.
                                  She does want to
sleep   with him,   her male friend, but I   know it's not   him
       but   his sex.
                 She has to remind herself that she's attracted to men so she won't be attracted to me.

E13.

Eventually he calms down.

                                                                I

suspect I am not welcome   but nobody tells me

        so.   Non-stop, drunken

babbling — nonsense —   I   hear the meaning,

                                                           so

subtle. But I choose to ignore

    the rejection

    of my gender.

E12.

                                         It floats up-river on the early morning mists —   her voice carries   well.   She loves him.

                            I want her to hold me and touch me and tell me that she loves me. But I can't

                                    be   male.

B5.

Words tumble out of my lips,
but I don't speak.

I don't have the courage to love her,
but, silent and drunk,
words slip anyway.

I should remain a secret,
I didn't want her laughing.

I thought she would have her male friend, first.

Still drunk, yet I get drunker,
and soon I can't drink anymore.

I hesitate to long to hold her.
Mask secure, I don't want to be without her,
and I know she'll find someone else to accompany her for…

I don't think thoughts like that.

93.

I keep my hands on something simple —
   a distraction.

Heart beating,
I open her hands:
   "I might be going too far."

She smiles:
"I find it interesting."

"Thank you."

61.

A falling sound.
Nobody hear it?

A soft voice…
staring could not have trapped any mouths
            into saying forced words.

She sits beside me and asks what I take to untie.

My faced singed red,
silently my embarrassment turns me.

Her smile unnerves me.
Shivering, pink-faced, I tell her.

I stand to leave,
she will accompany me.

Parting on the condition that she'll want
            our next encounter to be waiting…

Excited and eager,
I am foolish.

Just Plain Queer

96.

I find it hard to concentrate.
The smell of her perfume floats.

I want her.

I try to stifle this urge,
but it won't be stifled.

The dim lights screen these emotions.

She laughs:
"I thought you might want to leave with me."

89b.

I watch.
It's time.
My belly flops.

I miss hoping to stop feeling.

"It's been awhile."
This tiny fib escapes.

90.

She doesn't let me wonder:
"I thought you would be interested."

I tell her I could consider her.

She suggests I should do oral — daring.

I dredge up the courage…

When I am done, I bite the back between my lips.

88c.

An older lady tickles me.
Too slowly.

I finally feel wet.

I have a cigarette, no meaningless words.

(I feel like screaming)

88b.

Discussing is too hard,
Her words sound sincere.
I assume she is lying from jealousy.

I'd do the same, to avoid impressing.

88.

Staring at the falling rain,
I halve my medications.

I can't get up the energy,
the morning after, to apologize.

Struggling to remember my last memory
of her holding me,
I still feel sorry for the tugging urge
that insists she had something other than comfort on her mind
when she comforted me.

(Such fantasies)

85d.

My belly flops:

hoping both
to get there before seeing her,
and to run into her on the way.

My wish comes true.

82b.

I take her hand
— the twitch of feeling in my fingertips
　　asks me to hold her —
I willingly oblige.
Her body,
a desire to hold.

34.

Pleasure from my lips.

faster and faster

The bed is hard.
Deep in this,
I come.

79c.

Deteriorated,
tipsy,
no longer embarrassing,
I listen eagerly, wanting to know my prof.

32.

Pleasure of her...
    her lips, her mouth.

I remember shaking.

64.

My fingers,
    (swallowing naivety)
follow the path of her.

I feel my body melt away from me.
She wants.

54.

Her face presses in,
my heart clenched,
how could I - recoiling at the sudden knot in my stomach -
stare at this young, cool, smiling face
and just let her go,
and live my life alone?

But, the flame is out.

94.

You think me strange since you allowed me to choose.
   Weirdly, this is somehow romantic.

*I have never understood why one would
kill something so beautiful.*
Sudden thoughts chasing through…

Struggling to hold off these thoughts,
the courage to leave her does come.

I don't really have to explain —
until I see the look on her face.

60.

We are to discuss —
   things.
How we're doing —
   a chance to talk.

She nods and smiles, appearing to like what we say,
but I don't say anything.

I withdraw from the conversation.
The memories run behind my eyes.
I can't beg.
The burning threatens to smother me.

My futile frustration caught up in her sea-green eyes.
She smiles and holds my eyes a moment longer,
puts her hand on my shoulder,
before walking off.

I watch her leave,
unable to ignore the
~~excuse~~,
memories.

The Rising

69b.

My mother passes.
My memory takes me across the country to see her.
I focus, determined, I must go back.

I am calm, oblivious, I can not feel.

I am ready.

Back against the wall, I watch the second hand swing,
and wait,
hands out.

72.

My eyelids squint.
My head pounding with my heart,
my body screaming for its fix,
I collapse, my head resting on the bathroom radiator,
and vomit.

I try to miss myself, but don't succeed.
I spit up liquid.
I pull myself, vomit and all, to my feet,
grab my precious bottles —

pills held tightly, I take my medication.

69.

I stretch out, to hell.
Inside my head - wooden.

The clouds passing above me, questioning me.
I imagine those faces, dark, attractive —
cold.

A conclusion, the curiosity:
to be naked, is bad.

Tits to the world.

37.

Bitterness
(narrow, stubborn)
will never slip away.

13.

It tickles nobody,
to be perfectly honest.
Family, friends - slip into the woodwork
when you don't care about the stigma.

17.

Voice it.

Shame is only because I forgot
pain makes me feel real,
sometimes.

75.

Controlled for much too long
— Two years? —
(It couldn't have been that long or I would have noticed.)

Lying thoughts soon pop and I know fear.

75b.

I am still a few minutes:
I stop at the intersection for
uncomfortable lightness, reassuring feelings, odd joy, and
invited smiling.

I wait a very long time.

40.

The vast space, inside.
I beg for it to end
but only more laughter
lands and burns and scars.

I long for cover and I shiver.
Almost free,
I wipe the sweat from my forehead.

66.

Just acknowledge things happen that we can't let ourselves understand.

Try to imagine being with somebody on a date — somebody like me.

80.

I fall into nothing.
Thought works to impose — presumptuous,
some awkward burden.

I am content
to hang,
still,
in the cold.

39.

ignore the numbing dulling fight for survival -
the onslaught which starts the second
I buckle
under the pressure
of
the world
won.
I am sane and strong
but I have lost.

E23.

        I
              dare call   God.
  I know   there are   things worse than
going quietly and silently
                        and
          alone.
         There must be a reason for
this
          emptiness.

The Rising

1.

What I am thinking
it's much too big
I am on my knees,
God's voice talking.

81b.

I stand, shivering slightly in the chill air.
She fills the silence with her plans,
how comfortable, how real.

E17.

                                                                                               I emerge,

          strange

     lost

             invisible.   .

             The streetlights

             have been waiting in front of

             the   night.

They singe my eyeballs.

55.

My lips against an empty coffee cup
I look closely in the mirror,
it's not my own expressions.
I close my eyes - out of my skin.

It takes me a moment to stuff myself back in.

Content, I ignore the bird outside my window.

About the Author

Suzan Digh was born, raised and currently lives in Eastern Canada. She has been writing in poetic form since childhood and uses journaling, poetry writing, and long walks in nature to maintain her mental health.